The Nursing Survival Guide

A poetic interpretation on the path of a nurse

by Jeseeka Gustave MSN, APRN, FNP-C

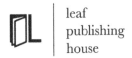
leaf
publishing
house

Dedicated to:

To my family, my roots, who helped me sprout wings,
My friends, the anchors, that kept me steady,
My coworkers, who nourished me, so I could grow,
To my sister Olivia, my inspiration, and hope.

I give thanks to:

the profession that gave me a voice
when I could no longer speak,
Gave me courage when fear kept me meek,
Ignited a passion to help those in need,
Provided me strength, when I became weak,
taught me the life lesson to put others first,
I give thanks to the profession, that made me a NURSE.

This is a guide on the path of a nurse,
It is not very angry, and I am not here to curse.
Maybe you'll laugh,
Or won't read it at all,
Maybe it'll captivate, and keep you enthralled,
But keep turning the pages,
Come on,
have a look,
This just might become your favorite guidebook!

how one becomes *a nurse*

So, you want to be a nurse?
Okay, grab a seat.
It isn't what the TV makes it cracked up to be.

It can be messy,
And it can be blue,
But it can also be meaningful for you.

You'll have your good days,
You'll have your bad,
sometimes you'll go home feeling quite sad.

But the work that you do,
And the lives that you change,
Make being a nurse,
The most rewarding of things.

Guide Tip: Nursing, a truly rewarding profession, will alter you in the most profound of ways. It will impact you to want and encourage change.

Are they the smartest of the bunch?
Quickest on their feet when in a time crunch,
Able to juggle five tasks at once,
Doing the job of many,
That is only meant for one.

Are they two parts sugar, that makes them so sweet?
A cup of surprise that makes them unique,
An unexpected delight that brightens your day,
And makes you feel better when things aren't okay.

What makes a Nurse?
It's nothing concrete,
define the nurse that you're going to be.
but first take that leap,
that scary first step,
when the question is,
"do you want to be a nurse?"
and the only answer is, "YES."

Guide Tip: What makes a nurse? If I had to guess, one-part savory, rich and sweet, another part spicy that adds a zing, and when you add it all up it's the most splendid thing.

You made the decision,
You handled with care,
You **decided to be a nurse,**
And the journey starts there!

Guide Tip: You will always remember the day you decided to be a nurse, because that is the day an idea took root, began to sprout, and a dream grew.

Where do you start,
And what do you do,
How do you get there?
And what to pursue?

What steps do you take?
And how do you choose,
The path that you know,
As **Nursing School!**

Guide Tip: There are multiple paths, but it all leads to ONE: the hardest academic years to come. Where tears will be shed, joy will be spread, and you will touch the lives of people you've only just met.

Do your research,
Find what fits,
Set expectations,
don't you quit!

Guide tip: Set expectations, create a timeline, and always, oh always, keep your goals in mind.

You have applied,
prerequisites are in,
Essay completed,
Application sent,
now you wait,
The decision,
Your fate,
The letter now open,
Destiny awaits!

Guide Tip: There is nothing quite like a **decision letter,** *one piece of paper that holds the future. One piece of paper that does not define you, and will never break you, regardless of its content.*

For those who didn't make it,
The decision was, **"We regret to inform."**
I implore you,
Don't give up,
Keep trying and apply once more,
For if you want to be a nurse,
And that is the road you choose,
"We regret to inform."
Should never discourage you.

Guide Tip: There is nothing more discouraging than a setback to a dream, but never forget, it is only a setback, and persistence is key.

You did it,
You made it,
The acceptance is in,
Enjoy it,
Embrace it,
The **hard work begins.**

Guide Tip: Hard work that includes sacrifice, determination, and commitment. Not the easiest of roads, but you must stay committed.

Inhale and exhale,
It's the **first day of class,**
Ease all your tension,
Let go, and relax,
It's just the first day,
It gets harder from here,
Express all your worries,
And voice all your fears,
They'll set expectations,
Go over the rules,
And you'll learn how to survive,
nursing school.

Guide Tip: How does one survive nursing school? Maybe with loads of caffeine, maybe with lots of prayers, or maybe through lack of sleep. Regardless of the answer, just try your best, work your hardest, and you'll succeed.

.

Bundles of note cards,
Pen stains on hands,
Pages and pages
Of nursing care plans.
Whispers of Patho,
Complaints of Pharm,
Sleepless nights,
Early morning alarms.

Guide Tip: Nursing school: Difficult, sometimes overwhelming, but certainly life-changing.

Key:

Patho - Pathophysiology

Pharm - Pharmacology

Two of the many classes taken in nursing school.

Our eyes meet,
we share a secret,
Inside jokes,
The chatter is frequent,
They tell us to hush,
The inseparable bunch,
Friends that study,
Nursing buddies.

Guide Tip: Nursing Buddies,
essential to nursing school survival.
They will make you laugh,
when you are about to cry,
they will make you stronger,
and urge you to try.

How do you study?
The night before,
Weeks of prep,
'Til you know
No more,
Pages of notes,
Fun little quotes,
Home alone,
With your books up close.
Maybe in a group,
learning something new,
Maybe to the music,
Moving to the groove,
What's most important,
Is you find your own tune.

Guide Tip: Dance to the beat of your own tune, find out what works, and what is opportune.

You prepared for this,
The **first exam,**
Hours of study,
The last-minute cram,
Relief as the test is underway,
Answers look familiar,
Just might get an "A."

Guide Tip: It's when the answers look unfamiliar, that you continue, make an educated guess, whisper a silent plea that you will pass this test.

The pack of students who **stick together,**
Birds of a feather,
in all kinds of weather.
Each one, tied to the other,
will survive if they help one another.

Guide Tip: Like a bird, you are a part of a flock. A group of people who are going through similar circumstances who just might have the same worries, fears, and emotions as you.
sometimes to survive and overcome,
one must remember,
it is better together,
than better alone.

Cup of coffee,
Bag full of books,
Rainbow of highlighters,
Notes in every nook.
Laptop on charge,
Pen marks on arm,
Bags under eyes,
PowerPoint slides,
Nursing school apparel,
Scrub sets that match,
Social media breaks,
Lecture hall naps.

Guide Tip: **Nursing school essentials as told by the survival guide:** *Coffee to start the day, and study breaks to keep you sane.*

You fall,
You stumble,
You want to give up,
Friends will cheer,
encourage,
And tell you, **"get up."**

Guide Tip: Nursing school is a lot of things- it can be frustrating, stressful, and it is easy to want to throw in the towel. I am here to tell you that there are those who are rooting for you, and if you fall, they will urge you to get up and keep heading towards the finish line.

The fundamentals,
the starting point,
You'll learn it in lab.
from textbook to practice,
to useful tactics,
the learning of hand-washing,
The starting of IVs,
the successful insertion of a Foley.
A few of the plenty,
and some of the many,
things you learn in lab.

*Guide Tip: **Nursing lab**, where you first start to learn the groundwork to a vast field of study. A vast field of study that is like an endless book just waiting for its pages to be discovered.*

Key:

IV - Intravenous (within a vein), nursing students learn to place IV lines on patients through which IV medications (medications administered to the vein) are given.

Foley Catheter: A urinary catheter placed through the urethra into the bladder to drain urine. Another skill nursing students are taught to perform is the insertion of a Foley Catheter.

Check a temperature-
warm or cold?
Feel a pulse,
fast or slow?
Oxygen levels are they low?
On their arm they will feel a squeeze,
As we get their blood pressure, please.
Respirations make sure you count,
take their pain into account,
Vital signs we have to get,
Before we go on to assess.

Guide Tip: Vital are the vital signs as they can tell us much about a person. Are they anxious, are they ill? If there's something wrong the vitals should tell. If they don't, hopefully the assessment will.

Inspect every area,
Palpate and feel,
Percuss tapping gently,
Auscultate to hear.

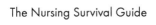

Guide Tip: These are the four essential techniques when assessing a patient, and it is all about using the senses. Sight and what you see, touch and what you feel, listen to what you hear.

Let's start with the head, ear, nose, and throat.
Don't forget the eyes, shine a light on them folks.
Shrug the shoulders, check the neck,
Time to go down to the chest,
take a deep breath,
Those lungs sound clear, now those heart sounds I hope I hear.
Lub-dub and there we go. Let's keep heading down below,
There's the abdomen, bowel sounds heard.
When you palpate, soft, non-tender is preferred!
Check the arms and legs, are peripheral pulses intact?
Reflexes active, ask about the urinary tract?
Any frequency, urgency, pain when they pee,
If it's a no, let's go down to the feet.
Wiggle the toes, flex each foot and extend,
Check all extremities, to rate muscle strength,
And evaluate the back, with a forward bend.
Throughout the exam inspect the skin,
for that is one of the places infection can begin.
observe their gait, balanced and steady?
are they oriented, alert, and ready?
once the examination is finished,
Jot down what you know,
Now you've done your **head to toe.**

Guide Tip: The head to toe assessment: what you see, and what you assess, can save the lives of those in distress.

Come on grab a kit,
Find an arm you can stick.
Look for a vein,
tie the tourniquet.
Steady the arm,
angle the needle just right,
Don't take too long,
That tourniquet's tight.
Have the hand make a fist,
Find a vein that is straight,
See that vein over there
Doesn't it look great?
Now, don't you wait,
Go for it!
Is that a flash of blood I see?
Advance the catheter,
Set that tourniquet free.
Secure it well,
Sign and date,
Now you have an IV in place.

Guide Tip: Never forget that **practice makes perfect,**
we each have our own timeline to learn how to do,
accomplish a skill, then perfect it too.

First, you add the assessment,
what they say,
And what you see,
Then formulate the nursing diagnosis,
What you believe the problem to be,
Next you start the planning,
How can I help with this problem today?
Follow-up with implementation,
You carry out your plan,
make sure everything is okay.
Finally, you evaluate,
Did your plan provide a fix?
And there you have it,
What the **nursing care plan** depicts.

Guide Tip: The nursing care plan depicts the plan of care but never forget how we care. We care with no reservations, or strings attached, without judgment, selflessly we act.

Once your clinical skills are proficient,
and check-offs are achieved,
simulations conquered,
is the moment you'll proceed,
to an unfamiliar venture,
within reach of your dream.

Guide Tip: To do is to learn, and to learn is to do. Execute the skills you have learned on real-life patients and continue to learn during **clinical rotations.**

The first day jitters,
The what if,
And what not.
I can't,
And have not.
Deep breaths,
And stay calm,
You will,
If you stay strong.

Guide Tip: **The first day jitters.** The nervousness because of
the unknown.
Will you remember things learned, or will you crash and burn?
No, with perseverance, you will excel and learn!

The first day of clinical **the professor says,**
"These are the rules to abide by,
Follow the example of the nurse to whom you are assigned.
Never do anything alone or without a guide,
If you have questions please ask,
You are in charge of what you learn,
Put yourself to the task.
Don't be afraid to get your hands dirty,
It can be scary, but we'll help with your worry."

Guide Tip: The age-old saying that you are in charge of your own destiny. Life only gives as much as you are willing to put in. So, put in your one hundred and ten percent and watch life take you to places you've never imagined.

The **nurse says to the student,**
"Do as I say,
Not as I do,
there is always time for question or two,
There is the textbook way to do it,
Or the nursing way to it,
Just follow my lead,
You'll learn what to do."

Guide Tip: It's simple, there is the textbook way and then there is the nursing way.

The **student says to self,**
Quietly, so no one can hear,
"You've got this,
You can do it,
Be confident,
You'll pull through,
Listen to the advice of others,
As they were once in your shoes."

Guide Tip: Never forget to listen. Listen to the guidance of those whose footsteps you follow. They have stood where you now stand. They have experienced your uncertainties and they understand.

"You're a student," they say,
"Well come on, I won't bite."
They'll joke and they'll tease,
And might give you a fright.
You'll be nervous with every little thing that you do,
And they might be there to reassure you.
You'll work very hard,
To please and to comfort,
And they might just laugh at your little blunders.
Your very **first patient,**
You'll never forget,
And when the day ends,
May they declare,
"you're the best."

Guide Tip: There is nothing like your first patient as a nursing student. You do everything you can to please, and when the day is over you would like to believe that you were the best student nurse you could be.

"I didn't expect nursing to be messy,
that I would have beds to make,
would be at the beck and call of others,
I thought I would have lives to save,"
The nursing student says in frustration,
For all who'd listen, to hear.
The nurse says in response,
"With every little mess,
every bed you make,
every call you answer,
That's a life you save."

Guide Tip: Nursing is built on monumental little things that make an everlasting impact. Making a bed, cleaning a mess, and answering a call light can truly make a difference for those who are sick in the hospital. Who knows, that call light you just answered might be another life waiting to be saved.

Key:

Call Light - A device that is at the patient's bedside that the patient uses to call for assistance from the nursing staff.

The clinical day has come to an end,
gather around as **post-conference** begins,
Where we discuss the day's adventures,
New lessons learned,
And new tasks conquered.
Tips and tricks that made us stronger.

Guide Tip: Oh the things you learn, and how they enlighten you. How they feed your enthusiastic mind with the nourishment of knowledge, leaving you eager and wanting more.

You will **rotate through many,**
And on some more than most,
You will find your greatest passion,
With confidence to boast,
You will learn all the quirks,
And tricks of the trade.
Discover new things day to day,
And whether it's Peds, Med-Surg, or ED
you might even have a knack for OB.
But the choice is yours,
follow your dream,
And with your passion help those in need.

Guide Tip: You will get a chance to get a taste of a few medical specialties during clinical rotations. Relish every moment, take it all in. Find the one that you most enjoy and can see yourself savoring in.

Key:

Peds - Pediatrics

Medsurge - Medical-Surgical

ED - Emergency Department

OB - Obstetrics

There is nothing quite like OB,
caring for expectant mothers to be.
What about the marvelous world of PEDs?
The work that you do, with the children you treat.
And maybe you'll get a chance to go to the ED,
Imagine all the unexpected things you'll see.
What if you get to explore critical care?
The critical thinking you'll need over there,
There is always Med-Surg,
A little bit of everything but **oh will you learn.**

Guide Tip: Med-Surg, Critical Care, ED, PEDs, and OB,
each one brings its own set of qualities,
but choose the one that excites you most,
keeps you guessing,
and has you engrossed.
Choose the one that brings a tingle
of passion to the soul.

Key:

Critical Care (ICU) - Intensive Care Unit

Maybe this journey wasn't for you,
And the path is slipping from the rearview.
You hear the whisper, "not cut out for this."
You hear the murmur, "maybe you should quit."
But you look ahead in a distance, not too far,
And you see your support system urging you on.
They are chanting, screaming, and jumping for joy.
And what are they chanting through all of that noise?
"Come on! let's do it.
Don't you quit,
You will be a nurse,
We are certain of this."

Guide Tip: Maybe you failed an exam or didn't pass a class. These things are setbacks, so take a step back, and come up with an action plan to get back on track. Most importantly remember when the thought comes to mind "maybe this isn't for me" there are those on the sidelines telling you that they believe. What do they believe in... you of course! If this is something you truly want, it is time that you start believing in yourself.

It begins in fall,
winter to spring.
Then there's summer
and the time in-between.
Exams come and go,
Rotations pass by slow,
'Til you're towards the end,
With a future to attend.
Time to prep for boards,
Graduation at your door,
The final practicum will commence
Soon **a new path will begin**.

Guide Tip: The first day seems like a lifetime ago, and the last day is about to arrive.

Cumulative,
Testing on everything you've learned.
To assess your readiness,
For the future you have earned.
The graduation exam,
The final scene,
One step closer
To your lifelong dream.

Guide Tip: The final scene, soon enough the curtain will close, you will take your final bow, and await the thunderous applause to follow. Some call it the end of the show, but I call it the beginning you have yet to know.

To the graduate

You have waited for this moment,
Where you will cross the stage.
Feelings of anticipation,
remembering the milestones you made.
The voyage it took to get here,
The doubts you never shared,
A future that's uncertain,
And the excitement that is there.
If I can impart wisdom,
With hope you won't forget.
From this moment forward,
Move forth with no regret,
As one of your greatest life's journeys,
You haven't lived it yet.
Embrace the life you're given,
Provide change through healing hands,
With every task be driven,
And know that sometimes things don't go as planned,
I expect that each and every one of you,
will take what you've learned and soar,
Onward you go, to see what life has in store.

Guide Tip: Congratulations! It wasn't easy getting here, and there were speed bumps along the way. Yet you have reached your destination, and what an accomplishment you have made.

You have survived
On to what's next...
that which is scary,
the licensure test.

Guide Tip: The licensure test will have you feeling like a bubble about to burst from anticipation and nerves. Anticipation because it is one of the road blocks that you have to hurdle over during the race to become a nurse. Nerves because the contents of this test are unknown, and the results of this test will determine a key aspect of your future. This is a race I hope you win, this is a race that I wish you the best of luck in.

Key:

The Nursing Licensure Test/Exam: Is an examination that nursing students who have graduated from nursing school must pass in order to be licensed as a registered nurse.

Each country has its own process. In the US and Canada nursing students must undergo the NCLEX: National Council Licensure Examination.

Take an intermission,
A break from the storm,
A moment of silence,
Before you experience the swarm,
Of job decisions,
And licensure prep,
Take **a moment for you,**
Before the next step.

Guide Tip: Self-care is the best care, it is important to take an intermission, before the transition, of making major life decisions.

Take a deep breath,
It's **just an Exam,**
Don't let it deter you from all of your plans,
Sure, it will determine your life long fate,
But take a deep breath,
Answer one, awaits.

Guide Tip: Deep breaths, a steady hand, maybe a prayer for luck. This is the moment that stands between you and your dream. This is the moment I hope you achieve.

I would like to introduce,
As you haven't formally met,
With greatest honor I present,
Registered Nurse
R-N.

Guide Tip: I would like to welcome you to the world of RN. We are a workforce of many, always ready to welcome more.

RN

Reliably Nurturing,

Resiliently Noble,

Relevantly Necessary,

Radiantly Nice,

Registered Nurse.

Guide Tip: Each year a new crop of registered nurses makes their debut. May we nurture them, provide them with strength, guide them with our knowledge, and with our aid may they flourish.

how one defines *a nurse*

You're **officially a nurse,**
The letters behind the name,
The hard work shown,
A profession you can claim.

Where to next on this wayward journey,
Off to beyond, and seize your glory,
Expand your horizons, and broaden your scope,
But first, take a moment,
And find yourself work.

Guide Tip: If you haven't already, get on it quick.
Look for a job and find the right pick.

Search high and low,
Far beyond or below,
Maybe around the corner,
Or simply down the road,
Maybe across the way.
Or in another state,

Search till you find,
With no end in mind,
The **job that will define,**
The nurse of your kind.

*Guide Tip: Search, and don't settle, because your first job will be
the groundwork, the building blocks to what builds you as a nurse,
and without sturdy ground,
one may crumble.*

Describe yourself in three words?
Passionate, motivated, and ready to learn.
What makes you a good fit?
Given a task, I won't quit.
why should we pick you for the job?
My goal is to save lives and never stop
And this aligns with the position you've got,
Whether you pick me, or the person up next,
I am grateful for the opportunity,
And hope that no one objects.

Guide Tip: You are an invaluable asset that would be a great addition to any team. Never forget this, and most importantly don't undersell your worth as you are the best product on the market.

We would like to **offer you a position,**
And we hope it's the first one you accept,
We offer many great opportunities,
And it is our deepest wish that you say yes.

Guide tip: The job offer, may it be the first of many, with plenty more to come. Unless of course you've found the right one.

I've been offered a position,
And I am inclined to say yes,
I can see growth in this position,
My response is, **"I accept."**

Guide Tip: The Acceptance - the decision wasn't made lightly,
you weighed out your pros and cons,
saw this as the first step to the future,
in a career that can be fairly long.

Dear New Nurse,

Welcome to a profession of many,
where you may be one of few,
to walk down this unknown path,
that I had the pleasure to walk once too.

The road up ahead is scary, filled with trials unforeseen,
But also filled with triumph, prosperity within your means.

Companion, I may never meet,
Comrade, I hope to one day greet,
Let me share the counsel that brought success to me.

May you **always be c**onfident, because in tough situations,
Confidence shows, and provides reassurance,
Even when unsure.

If ever overwhelmed, you are not alone,
Ask for the aide of others, and this will drive you home,

Always stand your ground, have faith in what you know,
Keep an open mind, as you will forever continue to grow.

My dearest new nurse,
In this path, I wish you well,
And it is my warmest wish,
In this path, you will not fail.

Guide Tip: My hope for you is that you never drown under your new role's sometimes-enormous expectations. I hope that you will always stay afloat, and if you feel yourself sinking, may you reach for aide and may it keep you whole.

Key:

ABC - Always Be Confident

I'd like to welcome you to the hospital,
Your new home away from home,
Many days will be spent here,
Through these doors, many have come.

We house those in need,
Those who are too sick to leave,
here for any, and every, emergency.
Open 24 hours a day,
Seven days a week,
Here in the hospital, we get no sleep,
We are glad that you could join us,
You are the backbone of this place,
It is our pleasure to tell you,
Welcome to your first day.

Guide Tip: The one place that is always open, and never closes its doors. Home to registered nurses, patients, and much more.

Time to go to the unit,
others call it the floor,
Where countless sounds ring,
Every corner there's a beep,
Anyone and everyone will peek,
When walking through those double doors.
Patient rooms are lined,
The nurses' station you'll find,
Your future habitat,
Can you imagine that?

Guide Tip: The **medical unit** *- many will walk through its doors, some with the intention to recover from illness, and some with the purpose to help those who are ill.*

You are new.
Newer than new,
Fresh, novice,
need guidance,
to breakthrough.

Guide Tip: With the help of a preceptor you'll make do.

A teacher that navigates,
Provides direction to the course,
The first of many friends,
A colleague, and a vital resource,
Assigned to assist,
In training, they persist,
They'll lead you right along,
Until you're set to move on,
On your own they watch you go,
When you're ready,
A **preceptor** knows.

Guide Tip: A preceptor, a guardian angel that guides you through the first of many ventures as a nurse. When you are primed and set for flight, they will tell you to spread your wings and fly.

This will be your constant,

For twelve hours on some days,

You'll even have the pleasure to work twelve-hour shifts

Three days straight.

Your coworkers will become family,

You'll learn the importance of team,

And at times you'll wonder why the call light always rings,

Bathroom breaks are a blessing,

When you're always on your feet,

And your patients are the ones you really need to please,

They say the heart of the bedside,

And the soul of patient care,

A **bedside nurse,**

With the motto to,

"take care."

Guide Tip: The bedside, the stomping ground for most nurses. Where twelve-hour days are most common, and chaos can implode at the drop of a hat.

The truth is simple,
With so much to discern,
You'll need support at every turn.
A guiding hand,
If only for a bit.
A short **orientation,**
I must admit.
A helpful transition,
Where you won't be alone,
A time for you to savor,
Cherish, and learn.

Guide Tip: You'll hear it often, which makes it true. Orientation is a moment for you. Where you can question, ask, inquire and learn, before you are set off on your own.

Before we move forward,
And get our hands wet,
Introductions are in order,
Your coworkers you haven't met.

Guide Tip: A different type of family, the type of family where every celebration requires a potluck, and on the toughest of days the motto is, "divided we fall, together we overcome."

In the case of an emergency,
I am the first one on the scene,
If you want compressions,
Most people ask for me,
For a patient in distress,
I am not too far behind,
I can detect,
When a patient will decline,
Some like to call me,
And most often do,
The nurse you need in an emergency,
Here to welcome you.

Guide Tip: There is always that one nurse who excels in an emergency, an adrenaline junkie with rapid response being their high. When a patient starts to crash, that's the nurse you need to ask.

If a call light rings you won't find me
For some reason, I am never there,
But if you were to ask,
I am off doing patient care.
And with all the care required,
I am too busy to be seen,
And most of the time
That happens to be
When the call light rings,
I guess they like to call me,
Although the name doesn't fit,
The nurse that never answers the call light,
But just between you and me,
The call light doesn't quit.

Guide Tip: The one nurse you like to call a magician, because when the patients call, they are never there. Oddly enough though, they are the first ones in the room handling patient care.

Some say I take frequent breaks,
I say that's not fair,
How can I work these long hours,
And not take a break here or there.
You might see me with coffee,
Or maybe in the breakroom,
But I am the only who'll ever say,
You need to take a break too.
So, come on
take a seat,
Let's have a little chat,
The nurse who takes frequent breaks,
Says sit back and relax.

Guide Tip: Twelve-hour days can be long, and you'll often hear nurses say they have not taken a break. I must commend the nurse who takes a break no matter how busy the day is because truth be told, those minutes of sanity where you can sit down and eat a meal among all the madness can really make for a better day.

I am most often overwhelmed,
And always on the go,
I find myself quite behind,
No matter how well the patient I know.
I question, and second guess,
They say I'm such a mess,
Disheveled they agree,
Help is what I need,
I am the nurse that's always behind,
But most helpful in a bind.

Guide Tip: The heart hurts for the nurse who is frequently behind because they just can't seem to get ahead. The heart also admires, because despite how far behind they are the nurse to consider a friend, for when they are not behind, a helping hand they will most often lend.

I never worry,
Quick on my feet,
I'm in no hurry,
While others run around,
I am calm, without a sound,
Chaos may ensue,
Panic may accrue,
But **nurse good under pressure,**
Never breaks down,
Will you?

Guide Tip: The one who stays calm during the storm is the one who will weather it through.

I've been here for years,
So, I know a thing or two,
They come to me for guidance,
I am the one they look too,
If there's a problem they can't solve,
There's an answer I will have,
If there's a dilemma I'm involved,
Through my experience I take charge,
The **senior nurse** with stories to tell,
Come to me if you need help.

Guide Tip: Respect the ones that say, "I remember back in the day." Let them impart their wisdom, and may you feed off their knowledge with the hope that it will help you grow.

Full of hustle and bustle,
There is no time to sit,
During this shift,
Things happen quick,
Appointments are pending,
Interruptions are made,
Management scurries,
With no occasion for delays,
Noise is surrounding,
Silence unfulfilled,
The day is filled with uncertainty,
And time does not stand still.

Guide Tip: **Dayshift** *- a great big juggling act, where you're expected to maintain balance through all the interruptions, unexpected delays, the sudden twist of events that daylight brings.*

I am just exhausted,
Up twelve hours of the night,
At the end of my shift,
I am sure I'm such a sight.
My shift isn't as bustling,
As the day shift might be,
But during the night,
is when confusion creeps.
Full moons are a worry,
Similar to Friday the thirteenth,
The night is full of superstition,
And a lack of sleep.

Guide Tip: **The Night Nurse**, *it takes a special person to work all hours of the night. As the night is unpredictable, filled with silence, but full of noise. Your greatest purpose is to help the patients sleep, in a place where alarms ring, confused individuals might scream, and medications need to be given at all hours, including when the patients sleep.*

Be careful,
I must warn you,
some nurses eat their young,
they devour,
shred to pieces,
leaving nothing but the bones.
It is tragic I tell you,
for they were once devoured too,
now they believe,
the cycle should continue,

But let us not be silent,
for this cycle we need to break,
for when **nurses eat their young**,
they scare the young ones away.

*Guide Tip: A word of caution to the new nurse, if you ever
encounter a nurse that eats their young.
A nurse that ridicules, and torments those who are new.
Remember, it is difficult for one to flourish when under strain,
it is hard for one to prosper when met with disdain,
and silence does nothing to break this revolving chain.*

A nurse isn't just defined by the registered in their name,
There's the **licensed practical nurse,**
Who is a nurse all the same,
Who carries out tasks,
And applicable skills,
Our comrade at arms,
Our companion in will.

Guide Tip: A nurse is... A nurse is many things, registered, licensed, certified. There is not just one role that delineates the position of a nurse, but multiple facets that structure, outline, and shape the sculpture, the masterpiece, the work of art that is... a nurse.

In highest regards,
With deepest respect,
With frequent encounters,
And the greatest effect,
A fundamental partnership,
An essential alliance,
Members of a team,
That requires compliance,
The oldest of friendships,
On similar ends,
That of **a nurse, and a physician,**
May a physician
be a friend.

Guide Tip: The oldest of friendships, two professions that work in partnership with one another. A physician and a nurse. While a nurse follows the orders of a physician, a physician follows the instincts of a nurse. Like any partnership, it only works if there is trust, respect, and in the case of a physician and a nurse, a mutual goal of taking care of the patient.

Is it others that define us,
As we follow in their place,
Do we take up their mantle?
Or make our own space.

Guide Tip: Let us never forget that people have influence, and you have the power to impact someone's life whether it is in a negative or positive light. Someone might be stirred by your actions to want to do grander, be better, or to follow in your footsteps. The truth is, the path toward greatness was sometimes built on the impact of others.

The preceptor says to the new nurse,
"We will go **down this road together,**
I'll teach you what I know,
We'll start slow and steady,
'Til you're ready to be on your own."

Guide Tip: Behind every great nurse is an amazing preceptor that helped mold, build, and shape. Behind every amazing preceptor is a great nurse that was ready to learn, eager to please, and would do what it takes.

The coworkers
say to the new nurse,
"We are grateful that you are here,
we hope that one day soon
you consider us home.
in us you have nothing to fear.
As part of our team,
only good days to come."

Guide Tip: We are grateful that you are here, a phrase that any new nurse would like to hear. As it is an exciting but frightful time, but the phrase "we are grateful" can ease the mind.

The new nurse says,
"time to take steps,
towards a direction
on my own,
a new role to play,
one that's not small,
one that is known,
where others stood before me,
and may I not linger behind.
Deep breaths,
And courage is key,
this is a time
I will define."

Guide Tip: Deep breaths are key,
Courage is all you need,
In order to succeed.
I hope the world sees all that you can be.
It is my wish that in faith may you dive,
Into the unknown in which you'll thrive,
Into a future in which you'll survive.

A good pair of scrubs,
Flexible and easy to clean,
For being on the run,
And unexpected spills you didn't see.
A reliable stethoscope
for when you really need to hear,
faint sounds that can save a life,
sudden changes you take in stride.
a comfortable pair of shoes,
that can withstand the test of time,
will keep you light on your feet,
for any emergency you should find.
A positive attitude,
for any given day,
amongst the disorder,
and amidst the disarray.

Guide Tip: **Nursing Necessities** - *scrubs that are good while on the go, a stethoscope that hears sounds the standard ears won't know, shoes that will keep you steady for twelve hours of the day, and a smile that will help you survive the disarray.*

Time to teach you **the basics**,
The groundwork to set you up,
The processes that will bring success,
As we have the pleasure to watch you progress,
Watch you shine on the brightest of occasions,
And never dim when things get dark,
Offer you direction and dedication,
To this new adventure, you are about to embark.

Guide Tip: Like a light bulb, shine bright for the world, provide light when things are dark, and never forget that sometimes the brightest of bulbs burn out.

We teach you about admissions,
How we get patients through the door,
What about discharges?
When the patient goes home once more.
Then their bedside report,
How long winded it should not be,
These are some of the things,
That **we have to teach.**

Guide Tip: Time for orientation, where you acquire the fundamentals to set you up for success. Where every occasion is meant for teaching, and you will learn things that can make the job easier.

First, we start with coffee.
Then off we go to bedside report,
Now we greet the patients,
Find out what they need,
And update the whiteboard,
Then we prioritize,
The important things that need to be done,
Maybe a break for breakfast,
With spirits refreshed,
Our day has begun.

Guide Tip: **How you start your day** *can define the rest of your shift. Some days start fast, and upbeat. other days start slow and sweet.*

Ask about the patient,
Orientation
Sense of mind,
Contact isolation,
How they walk?
Are they kind?
IV line?
What they do,
When they go.
Can a bedpan do the trick?
will they use the urinal?
Skin issues,
Any bedsores,
Discharge plans,
Headed out the door?
Don't ask too much,
But enough so you know,
Just how patient report goes.

Guide Tip: **Patient Report,** *keep it short and simple to get the necessary information in hand. It can be a short little recap of the twelve hours that might not have gone as planned.*

Greetings are in order,
Introductions should be made,
State your name
And purpose,
You are their nurse today.
Tell them of your intentions,
That for twelve hours you'll be here,
Ask them to call for assistance,
As you are always near.

Guide Tip: That first introduction, that initial greeting, does make an impact. Therefore, smiles are in order, a positive attitude we should see, and the only question to ask,
"is there anything you need?"

Partners in crime,
Attached to the hip,
A glorious device,
By your side, it sits.
Drawers full of pills,
Water pitchers filled,
Alcohol pads,
Saline syringes had,
Rolls from room to room,
Off you see it zoom.
Some call it a COW,
Others say WOW,
For a nurse it is ideal,
The **W**orkstation **O**n **W**heels.

Guide Tip: **W**orkstation **O**n **W**heels *(WOW) or for a lack of a better term* **C**omputer **O**n **W**heels *(COW). Just like a dog is man's best friend, a workstation on wheels is a nurses' favorite companion. And when choosing any favored companion, you must pick one that is reliable, efficient, and won't let you down.*

Go from patient to patient, room after room,
Start your AM medications, then comes afternoon,
If you work in the evening,
There's PM med pass,
and if you work in the night,
bedtime pass is last.
Make sure it's the right patient,
go over the meds,
is it the right drug?
right dose,
double check.
what route does it go?
and what time should it be?
open the meds,
and if there is a question,
you shall teach,
once all meds are swallowed
you are on to the next,
medication pass
you attempt to perfect.

Guide Tip: Perfection with medication administration, - is there such a thing? You are bound to mispronounce, experience a malfunction, or maybe even drop a medication. Mistakes happen even in the most perfect of scenarios. The best advice I can give is to be well prepared, have a general overview of what medications you are about to give, and fingers crossed with hopes for no spills.

Transcribe,

type,

paper to pen,

never forget to **document**,

Tell us what happened,

what did occur,

for if it is not written,

there is only your word.

Guide Tip: Let it be known that your words do carry weight, but documentation carries its weight in gold. For if it is not written others can say it wasn't done.

Time for our welcome,
The moment we say hello,
It's often frightening,
Being admitted to the hospital.
We get them comfortable,
Orient them to the floor,
Ask what brought them in,
Through the hospital's front doors.
Find out a little history,
And understand that they're scared,
it is now our job,
To provide them comfort and care.

*Guide Tip: **The Admission,** one of the first encounters the patient will have with the nurse. Expect that the patient might be scared. What they thought would be a quick trip to the emergency room turned out to be an overnight stay in the hospital. The one thing you can do to ease their discomfort is tell them of your presence and inform them that you are a resource upon which they can rely on, a hand they can hold, and a shoulder that they can lean on if ever they feel alone.*

Calling the doctor,
Oh, what a task,
Have your facts ready,
They'll be sure to ask.
I'm sure you are nervous,
will stumble on words,
Don't want to sound,
unwise, or absurd.
You want to sound intelligent,
Respect you will earn,
But let's not forget,
The patient's the concern.

Guide Tip: As a new nurse, calling the doctor about a patient concern can be scary. Hate to admit it, but doctors can be intimidating, and the saying goes "don't page me unless it is an emergency." I have a saying- If you have a feeling, a concern about a patient that won't go away, paging the doctor can't hurt. I would rather page and it be a false alarm than to not page and it leads to patient harm.

In the case of an emergency,
Don't panic,
Don't stress,
Hold your composure,
For the patient in distress.
Life hangs in the balance,
You've been trained for what to do,
Jump into action,
Call for help
To defuse.
Don't lose focus,
Have the patient in sight,
The only goal in mind,
Is to save a life.

Guide Tip: In the case of an emergency the patient is in fright, they look to the nurse for a calming sight. Don't let your apprehension or panic show, because the patient will feel it, they will know.

Time for goodbye,
the moment to part ways,
the road to recovery,
the end of their stay.
Maybe they are healed,
and headed home,
maybe it's terminal,
where comfort roams,
No matter the outcome,
best wishes we give,
and hope in their departure,
a healthy life may they live.

Guide Tip: Who doesn't hate goodbyes and a **discharge** *is the goodbye of medicine. Your time with the patient has ended, and maybe they are headed home or off to the unknown. You might have known them for two seconds, three whole days, or the majority of their stay. Regardless, there is a connection, and it is hard to see them go. If they are ready for discharge it is their time to take a different road. I can only hope that road is headed home.*

First, we started you off at one patient,
And once you were comfortable
We went up to two.
Got your bearings,
Then there were three.
You're a pro,
Now up to four,
Understaffed, you're at five,
Callouts happen,
you're at six.
Time passes by,
You're running the show,
With little assistance,
You're on your own.

*Guide Tip: The orientation of a new nurse is a steady process of taking care of one's own patients. Started off at one, then go on to two, but it depends on where you work that determines what a full patient load is to you. **Slow and steady** wins the race, take your time and go at your own pace. Even when you are ready to be on your own, you will still have much to learn.*

You've had a taste of the foundations,
That will only help build you up.
You've acclimated to your surroundings,
Are still a novice,
But proficient enough.
You continue to learn as you go,
from this moment forth you will be on your own,
But in truth, and in fact you are **never alone.**

Guide Tip: If only one thing resonates in your heart and mind through this whole process let it be this, "you are never alone." You are not a solo soldier, but a part of a large and powerful army that you need only turn to when you seek support.

Is it through flaws,
weaknesses,
one's character or traits,
through moments,
actions,
that help create.
The whole individual,
The trusted human being,
That has the pleasure of
Taking care of me.

*Guide Tip: What is it that helps create or define the human being that has the honor of taking care of the sick and the ailing? I believe that there is nothing definitive, each person has their own uniqueness that brought them on the **path of healing** the sick. A path that crosses with many and intertwines with most.*

To answer the question,
The inquiry of sorts,
What defines us,
And makes us more,
The answer is simple,
But difficult as well,
Truth be told,
It's hard to tell,
Maybe it's circumstances,
People we meet,
Maybe through experiences,
Or problems we greet,
Maybe you have yet to define,
The role that you play,
In this single lifetime.

Guide Tip: The question should not be what defines us, but what defines you? Truly, the response is you define yourself. With this simple, yet complex answer, we start to understand **what defines a nurse.** *Each nurse determines what type of nurse he or she will be. Maybe they will be the nurse who is always in a bind, or maybe the nurse who never has the time. Just know that once you define, it can be hard to redefine, the role that you might play in this once and a lifetime.*

Training wheels off,
And on may you soar,
On your own now,
To learn and explore.

Guide Tip: Like a baby bird set to take flight, you are unsure. What if you don't soar up high but fall down below. It is scary to fly solo to unchartered territories and unforeseen horizons, but it is also thrilling to start your solitary adventure. So, spread your wings, and off you go, to start a journey you can now call your own.

how a nurse **conquers and refines**

I've held the hands of dying patients,
Seen tragedy at my feet,
Held together those who suffer,
And in my heart, I silently weep,
For those who will never know justice,
The young ones who died too soon,
The elderly who have suddenly forgotten,
All that they once knew.

I carry the strength of others,
As they have no more strength to give,
In their weakest moments,
It is my hope they have the will to live.

Compassion at my fingertips,
What stands between life and death?
A patient's greatest supporter,
Your nurse,
With the simple question of,
"How can I serve you best?"

Guide Tip: The hands of a nurse and the wounds they have tended, the eyes of a nurse and the things they have seen, the heart of a nurse and the people it's mended, the strength of a nurse that never gives up.

May you flourish in uncertain circumstances,
May you never waver in a difficult decision,
May you always go with your gut feeling,
May your intentions be to provide healing.

Guide Tip: May you always provide healing, and may your intentions be to do no harm.

There are jitters and nerves,
Doubts and concerns,
As you mark the footsteps
Of being on your own.
You're afraid to let go,
Of the **hand that took hold,**
That guided you through,
To what was fresh and new.
But the hand you release,
Walk forward to meet,
The endless possibilities,
That now stand at your feet.

Guide Tip: Even after you let go of the hand that guided you, taught you and reassured you, it will always be there to continue to provide comfort, support, and encouragement. Never be afraid to turn towards it, grasp it, or take hold of it when you need help.

You now have your own team,
Where you run the show,
Patients under your care,
As you develop your flow,
Conquer unforeseen problems,
Refine tricks that are old,
Work easier indeed,
Not harder is the decree.

Guide Tip: **Work smarter, not harder,** *and find the tricks of the trade. As these tricks, when in a dilemma, can come to your aide.*

Today I am your nurse,
For better or for worse,
Through sickness,
When health fades,
Through darkness,
and days of grey,
Through light,
In enlightening times,
To fight,
When the fight,
Your will can't find.

Guide Tip: You enter into a silent vow when you take a patient under your care. You vow to care for them for better or for worse, through sickness when health fades, and sometimes 'till death do us part.

Hour one: day shift or night shift to come,
Hour two: patient report to review,
Hour three: medication pass to get to,
Hour four: doctors' orders to go through,
Hour five: insulin shots before lunch,
Hour six: take a break, with snacks to munch,
Hour seven: more medications to do,
Hour eight: missing meds, nothing new,
Hour nine: discharges, look at the time,
Hour ten: admissions is what it brings,
Hour eleven: time to wrap up things,
Hour twelve: off to report we give,
And it is the end of our **twelve-hour shift.**

Guide Tip: There are 24 hours in a day, and a nurse will spend twelve of those hours at work. During that time period anything and everything can happen, the day can be bad or good, time can go slow or swift, during a twelve- hour shift.

Key:

Insulin - A hormone that regulates the amount of glucose in the blood. It is used as a medication to treat high blood glucose levels in patients with diabetes.

A nurse will encounter,
The many, but different,
The similar, yet the same,
The diverse, but unique,
The kind, grateful, and sometimes their mean,
the very many patients a nurse will meet.

Guide Tip: **Patients***, each with their own story, and particular set of traits. With one thing that connects them - the nurse; that heals, cares, and advocates.*

Highly displeased,
And ready to leave,
You beg and plead,
But they don't concede,
You advise them of the risks that leaving pose,
Against **M**edical **A**dvice is how it goes.
They made their choice,
You must respect,
You say goodbye,
But with great regret,
You'll see them soon,
For truth be told,
Health declines,
When sickness holds,
With deepest fear,
And greatest hope,
May healing spark,
And may they cope.

*Guide Tip: **Patient AMA**, is one you'll encounter often. They are not satisfied with the care they receive, hard to please, and eager to leave. They are the ones who need care, and it is for us to urge them to get care, if not here than elsewhere.*

They tell you no,
That they refuse,
don't see the purpose,
And what's the use,
You explain the benefits,
Expound on their care,
But they still go home,
And don't adhere,
And now they're back,
Things are worst,
Noncompliant is the word,
You educate to reach,
You emphasize and preach,
You hope they take heed,
Of the words that you teach.

Guide Tip: **Patient Noncompliant** - *None too compliant with care, you can teach and preach but it is up to the individual to open their ears, and let your words reach.*

Unbearable it is,
It aches and burns,
It's sharp and constant,
An excruciating concern,
Nothing makes it better,
And everything makes it worse,
Begging for relief,
Reaching out to feel at ease,
Hope that they'll recover,
Worry that things won't be the same.
Will they live life in persistent pain?

Guide Tip: **The Patient in Pain** - *one can't pretend to know or truly understand the pain that someone else goes through. We can get them calm, maybe ease their aches, and try to have them understand their pain might not go away. But they will withstand, they will survive, and we will get them to a place where they will still feel alive.*

The itch they can't scratch,
The constant fix,
Will do anything and everything,
To get their kick,
To feel the high,
The fatal dose,
When they withdraw,
Death comes close,
Tremors and shakes,
Life hangs in the wake,
They have their need,
but you wish they'd get clean.

Guide Tip: **The Patient with an Addiction** - *When there is a craving for something damaging, when nothing can satisfy the hunger except the thing that brings you most harm, then you are looking at the face of addiction. A face that you should never judge, a face to which you should offer assistance if they are ever ready to embark on the path of sobriety.*

Things are forgotten,
Memories slip,
Accidents happen,
An unintentional trip,
Frequent falls,
Assert that they have a grip,
Can make their own decisions,
Independently, can they live?
Pleasantly confused,
You are there to assist,
But they will insist,
They can handle this.

Guide Tip: The Confused Patient (pleasantly so), as we age things are forgotten, and memories slip, but we still want to maintain our independence. It is important to know that the power to make decisions for oneself is something that no one wants taken away. So, do your best to give them some sense of control, but safely and carefully is the goal.

Part of the family,
As if the hospital's home,
They spend more time here,
Than they do on their own.
All efforts are made,
To discharge them safe,
Help them manage their care,
And send them on to their place,
But they bounce back,
Sicker than before,
No shelter to hold them,
Vulnerable and alone,
The frequent flyer,
The one we all know,
The one when they're gone,
Is the one that we mourn.

Guide Tip: The frequent flyer is a recurring character that you see often, but not everyday, that you grow accustomed to and are saddened once you finally part ways.

The innocence,
The laughs,
When sick,
Things are sad,
The joyful youth,
a playful view,
full of life,
and endless smiles,
but it aches,
to see a s**ick child.**

Guide Tip: The sick child - there is nothing more disheartening than seeing a sick child. Instead of laughs, there might be tears, for someone so young to be so ill. Therefore, bring them joy, and try for smiles, provide them with comfort through these trials.

New life they bring,
An unexpected change,
The miracle of nature,
The nurture it rings,
The expectant mother,
The glow you will find,
For precious life,
They carry inside.

Guide Tip: The Expectant Mother, who carries the future of generations. At her most vulnerable state, we urge her with each passing breath to let new life make way.

"How can I care for this patient?
When appalling acts they have done,
appalling acts that cannot be undone,"
The nurse questioned and inquired.
The seasoned nurse responds,
"It is not for us to judge revolting acts,
Deeds that were done that cannot be taken back,
For once a patient walks through those doors,
Sins we must forget,
As an oath we swore,
Equal care to every patient,
Equal care, compassion, and dedication."

Guide Tip: In this profession, you will encounter people who have done unspeakable things. It will be difficult to swallow but remember, it is not for a nurse to judge based on past misconduct, current crimes or deeds, it is for us to help those who suffer, despite their misdeeds.

A shoulder to cry on,
A hand to hold,
An ear to listen,
For tales untold.
A smile awaits,
In difficult times,
A calming presence,
You will always find,
An oath taken,
A promise fulfilled,
Take care of our patients,
And take care we will.

Guide Tip: A pledge most promising, an oath not easily forsaken, to upkeep lives that have yet to be taken. With an end that is not in sight, a vow is made to bring comfort to life.

How do we conquer the path we are in?
Keys to the trade that help us make sense.
We prioritize with importance,
And delegate as one,
And appreciate those around us,
For all that they've done.

Guide Tip: Prioritize what's most important, delegate when tasks overwhelm, appreciate every moment, and every person that gave help.

What's most important?
Who should be seen first?
Prioritizing is how this works,
Emergent to urgent,
To that can wait a bit,
To finally reaching the last on our list.

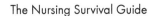

Guide Tip: You start with the ones that are most at risk, and end with the ones who need a quick fix. From the major emergency, to the minor stress, prioritizing can lead to the conquer of success.

A great many things to juggle,
With only two hands in place,
It is moments like this,
That we **delegate.**
Assign tasks to others,
as they undertake,
to help alleviate,
the duties that wait.

Guide Tip: You are part of a team, one piece of a whole, where all parts should work as one. Divvy up assignments, coordinate to get things done. You are one of many and are not the only one.

Never forget those around,
That assisted without a frown,
Stood beside when things went down,
Lifted a finger without being asked,
The ones to **appreciate,**
As they have your back.

Guide Tip: Value the ones who provide support, because in a field filled with unexpected turns, and forks in the road. It is good to get assistance wherever that road may go.

Anxiety as the load piles on,
Pressure with each second lost,
Tension,
Overworked, and overwhelmed,
Hesitation,
With no one to tell.
Concern as we count the minutes down,
We yearn for,
The hours to pass us by.
Our heart races as
We are unsure,
The day ends,
Can we continue to endure?

Guide Tip: In this high-stakes job, anxiety is an emotion a nurse will experience. It can overshadow, leave you out of breath, and have you overcome with stress. You are one person that is taking care of a life in its most vulnerable time. A heavy burden to carry, as so much can be on the line. So, I ask you to pace yourself, sit down if you need to, breathe in and out, and voice any issues. Unburden your load, and remember you are not alone, as others can help you, if you should condone.

Watch what you touch,
Be careful what you breathe,
Cover your mouth for any sneeze,
Gown and gloves,
Mask in place,
Universal precautions every which way.
Protect yourself,
And others too,
by obeying **precautions,**
You keep bacteria few.

Guide Tip: Protect your patients and protect yourself by doing something as simple as washing your hands. Sometimes the smallest of things are the ones that can do the most harm, and the things we can't see can be a danger to us all.

It's difficult to control,
When sick and ailing in bed,
The body will unroll,
The irritant it needs to shed,
Maybe it's a fever,
that will have them drenched in sweat,
Maybe it's the stomach,
That will have them quite upset.
They couldn't reach it fast enough,
Their body gave release,
There was such a **mess,**
It made them feel ill at ease,
They felt such embarrassment,
But they were met with smiles,
And the nurse simply said,
"Let me get some towels."

Guide Tip: Nursing can be quite the mess as you are dealing with fluids coming out of every orifice of the body, and it can be hard to control when sick. There will be unexpected projectiles, moments when patients couldn't make it to the bathroom and accidentally went on the floor. The patient might feel embarrassed, and it will be up to the nurse to reassure.

The skin is fragile,
It breaks,
And burns,
It scars,
And infects,
It bruises,
And bleeds,
can be wounded,
very deep,
to heal,
is to dress,
the **wound** that weeps.

Guide Tip: The skin is fragile, and when broken, sometimes hard to repair. But is also tough, and our coat of arms. It is our first layer of defense when the world means us harm.

Bedbound,
rarely moves,
Contracted,
Incontinence spews.
Skin impaired,
High risk,
total care,
to assist.

Guide Tip: The total care patient relies on the nurse to move, to turn, and to feed. They are dependent for most of their needs. They did not ask for the circumstances they are in, but are grateful for the care that you bring .

Bony prominences,
Stayed in one spot,
redness present,
hope it's not.
does not blanch,
identified as such,
Pressure Ulcer,
hard to the touch.
skin break down.
We must turn every two,
float the heels,
and assess the tissues.

Guide Tip: The Pressure Ulcer, proof that just enough pressure on one spot can cause breakdown, and breakdown takes healing, and healing takes time.

There are not enough words,
For me to fully express,
My gratitude,
And utmost respect,
To signify the importance,
Of the role that you play,
And how much your words,
Really hold in weight,
The commitment you give,
The difference you make,
There is no greater aide,
Than a **CNA.**

Guide Tip: **C**ertified **N**ursing **A**ssistant, *Patient Care Assistant, or Nurse's Aide. CNA, PCA, and NA. There is no greater support to a nurse, and like every support system we must commemorate, appreciate, and recognize their efforts. For where we would be, and what would we do, without our CNA.*

Have you **got the hang of things?**
Know your way around the block,
Built a routine,
Efficient like a clock,
Have you learned the tricks?
And how to make them stick,
Fine-tuned your methods,
And finally, it clicked,
Are you becoming an expert?
Not so novice and new,
Are you finding that this is, in fact?
The job for you.

Guide Tip: You've had a bit of time flying solo, so we are here to see how do you do? This is a moment to express frustration, or if this is a profession you can continue to pursue.

This is the nurse,
here to **check in,**
to let you know,
I'm getting the hang of things,
There have been slip-ups,
Mistakes have been made,
But things have been learned,
And lives have been saved.
It goes without saying,
not at all with dismay,
this is a profession,
I will continue to praise.

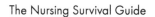

Guide Tip: The check-in, the moment you self-evaluate how things are going. Reflect on mistakes, rejoice and acknowledge, and look forward to all the feats you have yet to accomplish.

We gather,
We hover,
We worry,
We hound,
We might be one,
maybe nobody found.
We support,
Provide strength,
We endure,
At arm's length,
We watch in agony,
What sickness brings.
We're concerned,
We take heed,
Of what death might conceive,
who are we you ask?
We are **the family.**

Guide Tip: The family the nurse will encounter, it is inevitable as everyone has a family in some shape or form. It is the bond that holds us together when sickness unwinds. It is not always blood that binds, but friendship that ties, and love that knots us all together, It loops and weaves, unbreakable in strength, this complex tapestry known as the family.

In this bed, you will not stay,
Build your strength,
As weakness preys,
Baby steps we must make,
Baby steps we will take,
One foot forth,
None foot back,
Look ahead,
Towards the **Recovery Track.**

Guide Tip: It is essential to encourage movement to a patient who was sick and previously bedridden. Weakness preys upon the sick. It can be hard to get up after being down and out. So, one foot forward and don't look back. Start with a step, progress towards a gait, and once you are steady revival awaits.

It's a sickness we can't see,
That creeps every so silently,
It is one that can be difficult to treat,
As the mind itself, becomes the disease.

Guide Tip: **Mental health and illness,** *there are those who find it hard to defeat because it is something they can't see. Then there are also those who find it hard to believe as they only consider what they are able to perceive. It does not matter what we cannot see, or what we perceive to believe. The truth is the mind can become the disease and it is up to us to support and treat.*

Their words **cast stones,**
And pierce the skin,
Reach the soul,
Impact and cringe,
Their taunts wound,
And cut the heart,
Break down to pieces,
Torn apart,
They feed off weakness,
Ambition they'll seize,
They build themselves up,
By others defeats.
A bully by name,
Character and creed,
A bully whose actions,
will not succeed.

Guide: Unfortunately, there are bullies - people who are not here to lift you up but to bring you down, A great adversary to themselves only. Do not take their words to heart or acknowledge their actions. For you know the potential you have and the skills you possess. Often times it is difficult not to hear the words of those who berate you and make you question your purpose in this profession. But please listen and hear these words: You are a great individual who decided to join the ranks of a profession that can save and change lives. You are remarkable, and resilient, never let anyone make you question your purpose on this path you have chosen.

Things went wrong,
Mistakes were made.
Life moves along,
As you have a **bad day.**
The pressure you felt,
The walls closing in.
You're out of breath,
When will it end?
You want to quit,
And head for the door.
Burst into tears,
You can't take anymore.
Stress overwhelming,
You're gasping for air
you feel yourself sinking,
When a hand pulls you up from despair.
A faint whisper in your ear,
"don't give up on this day.
Stay strong fellow comrade,
And let tomorrow make way."

Guide Tip: As a nurse, a bad day you cannot avoid but a bad day will not destroy. A bad day is like a tunnel shrouded in darkness, with no glimpse of sunlight in sight. It is up to the weary traveler to step forward and journey towards the light. You are the author of each day in your life and how your day turns out, well, that is up to you to write.

There is no money in the cure,
But profit in the disease,
a statement made,
that does not appease,
As the poor suffer,
Take care of the rich,
for they can truly afford it,
so a price tag is placed,
On that which should be priceless.
Force to fight,
but won't be held silent,
for it is our right,
our purpose,
our plight,
affordable care,
for every single life,
it is a topic that scares,
that should only be fair,
we often despair,
known as **healthcare.**

Guide Tip: Let's take a moment and talk about health disparities. How not everyone can afford the basic human right of affordable healthcare. How part of the world suffers, and the other part it is a universal standard, reasonable care to all. The only thing that is fair is affordable healthcare, as a high cost on ones health and life, is the most displeasing and disagreeable sight.

Jeseeka Gustave

There is no "I" in it,
Not a solo act,
A collaboration,
With greater impact,
Different parts,
That combine as one,
Common goal,
To overcome,
United they stand,
Divided they fall,
Held in esteem,
We call them the **team.**

Guide Tip: Think of the bees who work in unison for a combined goal and create the sweet sustenance that is honey. Now think of the medical team who works in harmony and through their mutual work provide wonders in the healing of the sick. The hard work of one person can make a difference, but the collective work of others can make a change.

To the Team: The major part of the whole, the missing piece
of the puzzle, the foundation to what helps us stand tall in
moments in which we waver.

Thank you to the TEAM

PT: Physical Therapy   MD: Medical Doctor
OT: Occupation Therapy   LPN: Licensed Practical Nurse
RT: Respiratory Therapy   CNA: Certified Nursing Assistant
RN: Registered Nurse   KT: Kinesiotherapy
NP: Nurse Practitioner   PA: Physician Assistant

Pharmacy
Psychiatry
Social Work
Psychology

Guide Tip: Each profession has its role, none too big or small. Like the parts of a well-oiled machine, machines at times malfunction due to errors with the smallest of nails and maybe the largest of cords. It doesn't matter the size of the role; it matters **the part you play.** *If you don't work in unity with one another and don't play your part, that well-oiled machine that once functioned so beautifully will break down.*

To **conquer,**
Is to practice,
Hard work to overcome,
It takes time and effort,
A difficult endeavor,
A battle not easily won.

To **refine,**
Is to fine tune,
Fix the wrinkles and the creaks,
A different perspective,
But sometimes change,
Is hard to concede.

Guide Tip: Not all things will be conquered, but small feats will be attained. Not everything needs refinement, some things should stay the same.

The patient to the nurse,
"Something is not right,
uneasiness has taken hold,
With a nagging feeling,
unsure of going home,
Uncertainty and doubt,
Concern has come about,
To you, I bear this truth,
And it's you, I hope will soothe."

Guide Tip: No one knows more about themselves than the actual patient, so the phrase "I don't feel well, I don't feel ready, or I don't feel right," should be taken seriously. Even when there are no obvious signs, heed the patient's warning because they have the eerie ability to foretell their future when it pertains to sickness. Always remember to look, learn, and listen when it comes to your patient, as this can start a conversation, that can help to understand the situation, that is the patient's concern.

A colleague says to the nurse,
"The patient's concern,
An unsettling decree,
unnerving declaration,
taken seriously,
mountains we'll move,
and battles we'll fight,
all to bring our patients' concerns to light."

Guide Tip: One of the biggest roles a nurse will play is that of an advocator. Their greatest cause is to defend, with all their might, until the end; the patient. For those without a voice, who are often weak, are those for which we should use our voice, it's for them we speak.

The nurse to the provider,
"I need you to listen,
I want you to know,
I have a **gut feeling,**
This patient should not go,
Something is not right,
This patient's unwell,
I have a strong intuition,
That has me compelled,
To share my worry,
My apprehension and fear,
As time draws close,
misfortune is near."

Guide Tip: It is knowledge and experience that fuels your gut feeling, that lights the spark that is instinct, and feeds the fire known as intuition. All of which burns brightly when a patient is not healing.

"HELP," a voice screams,
"The patient can't breathe."
Next, we hear the scurry of feet,
The crash cart retrieved,
As its wheels slightly screech,
Code Blue it would seem,
Unconscious at the scene,
No pulse to detect,
Compressions to the chest,
At a rate of,
thirty then two breaths,
code team takes charge,
fast and swift,
by and large,
act quick,
a life to save,
unresponsive,
all we gave,
"time of death,"
Words we hate.

Guide Tip: The code, a tug of war between life and death. Where there are those who spectate and cheer for life, there are others at the end of the rope on each side. One side pulls with all their might for life renewed, and the other side filled with unknown forces tugs for death's pursuits.

The family weeps,
As eternal sleep
A loved one keeps,
It is **all who grieve,**
as tears slide silently,
Upon our cheeks.

Guide Tip: It is for us to grieve, sometimes silent so quietly, for a life taken too soon, even the anticipated death, we will say goodbye, as we lay them to rest.

Rest in peace friend,
To softer shores,
With calmer waves,
fruitful lands,
and blissful days,
Rest at ease friend,
To starry nights,
With nature's gaze,
Filled with love,
and warm embrace,
Safe passage on your journey,
No suffering filled with pain,
We send you off in peace,
to one day meet again.

Guide Tip: Death is sometimes inevitable with sickness. Life slips away, hands to hold as we pray, and we watch as the last breath a patient takes. It is hard when a life progresses on to the next, but to stay strong is to ease that life to a peaceful rest.

To the Nurse,

Who bears a great responsibility,
But does so selflessly.
Thinks of the plight of others,
Does not handle a life carelessly.

Wipes up tears filled with pain,
A shoulder to lean on,
One so humane.
Hard to direct gratitude
When words do no justice
to share in our thanks.

But to the nurse
We will always remember,
For they were the hand that guided us home,
The angel that laid us to rest,
The companion that shared in our worry,
The guide that helped healing progress.

To the nurse,
We express appreciation,
Thankfulness to their devotion
To lives of strangers
They made feel like a friend,
We are your patients,
Here to say thanks.

Guide Tip: Appreciation, it may not always be conveyed into words, but it is an unspoken truth that can be felt as if engulfed in a snug embrace. It is the understood silence that echoes the words **"thank you."**

It is time for the end,
The conclusion,
The curtain to close,
The intention was to motivate,
Inspire,
fill with hope.
encourage
and inform,
on the life of a nurse,
no desire to offend,
through these rhymes or words.
May you feel content,
As this story comes to a close,
Thanks for taking this journey,
And having a look,
to what one would hope,
is now your favorite guidebook.

Guide Tip: Heavy is the heart, that carries the burden,
of voicing the phrase, **"The End"**

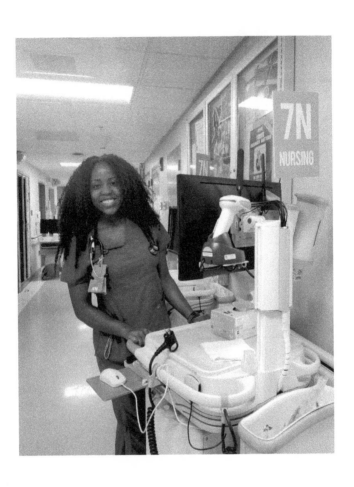

Jeseeka Gustave is a board-certified advance practice registered nurse, Daisy Award Honoree, and creator of the blog Confessions of a Nurse and Writer. She obtained her Bachelor of Science in Nursing from the University of Florida and her Master of Science in Nursing from the University of South Florida. After spending five years as a bedside nurse, she earned her certification as a nurse practitioner and was inspired to write about her nursing experience through her favorite literary avenue ~ poetry.

The day she left the bedside,
Was the day the words flowed through,
It was the moment she decided to honor
the nursing profession.

From a poetic point of view.

If you can't find Ms. Gustave traveling the world, writing on her blog, or taking care of her patients, then you can follow her on Instagram @nursepractitionerjess.

ISBN: 9781916309852